Clean Eating

A beginner's guide to eating clean, avoiding toxins, and feeling great, including recipes

I0423366

By

Faye Froome

Contents

Introduction

Thanks for buying this guide on Clean Eating.

I have produced this guide for people like myself whom yearn for healthy unadulterated food that modern life seems to have taken away from us.

Food we can rely on to be fresh and as free from toxins as possible. Today much of our food is mass produced in factories and sold in large stores for our convenience.

This convenience comes at a price. The foods we consume on a daily basis are designed to have a long shelf life in order to maintain your local stores profits. To aid the longevity of this food, it's pumped full of toxins in the form of salt, sugar and other chemicals.

The horsemeat scandal that rocked Europe a few years back is testament to how this type of processed food can be full of all sorts of things we neither want nor need in our food.

The obesity and health crisis that is swamping the western and developed world is largely down to the sugar, fat, and salt laden convenience food we consume far too much off.

The concept of clean eating dates back to the 1960's and is at the start of 'The Natural Health Movement'. This movement was originally founded with no thought as to the health and nutritional benefits of eating, instead it was based on protesting the societal pressures to dismiss the traditional mealtime routines and use convenient processed foods instead.

Despite the reasons behind the original clean eating diet, those within the fitness industry recognised the health benefits of eating clean food and before long the regime was being embraced by body builders, athletes and gym goers.

The physical and mental improvements being experienced by those actively eating clean did not go unnoticed and, as the interest in health and wellbeing increased throughout society, it did not take the media long to pick up it.

The labelling of this eating regime as a 'Clean Eating Diet' ensured it would quickly become the next big thing in eating and was adopted by many throughout mainstream Europe and America.

When people talk about the 'Clean Eating Diet' they are often met with looks of confusion, because it sounds like a complicated eating regime and many people assume it is just another fad diet that won't work.

It is, in fact, very simple once you understand it and this book has been written to help you do just that. It will also show that Clean Eating is just about the type of food you eat rather than a short term diet designed to lose weight fast or detox yourself.

Some of the most common questions regarding Clean Eating are listed below and all will be answered within the pages of this book.

- What is Clean Eating?
- How does it Work?
- Can it be Easily Maintained?
- Is it Suitable for Everyone?
- Is it Affordable?

I hope you enjoy trying out the recipes contained within and have fun experimenting with them using different herbs and spices.

The health benefits of putting natural ingredients into your body will have you feeling amazing in no time.

You will be stunned at the results.

Thank you for buying this book.

What is Clean Eating

Clean eating is based on one fundamental rule: Do Not Eat Processed Food!

This means consuming only 'Real Food'.

- **Real Food:** Single ingredients which contain no added chemicals
- **Processed Food:** Chemically processed foods which are manufactured using refined ingredients and artificial substances

While this sounds like a very simple concept, it can take some time getting used to because, as a society, we have become adept at choosing the easy option when it comes to our diet.

A combination of our busy lives and the bombardment of information that tells us cakes, carbohydrates and all manner of other foods are bad for us, has got us reaching for the ready-made foods provided by the food industry rather than preparing our own meals with real fresh ingredients.

Changing this mindset is the biggest obstacle when it comes to converting to a clean eating diet, but a little perseverance for a few weeks and this natural way of eating soon becomes the norm. In the end you won't even realize you are making clean eating choices!

Eating clean can be time consuming until you get into the swing of it on a regular basis because it requires time spent preparing and cooking your ingredients, something many of us are not used to, but there is no reason why some foods, such as curry, shepherd's pie and casseroles cannot be made in larger batches and frozen for consumption on another day.

There are also no restrictions on the type of food you can eat. If you want cake, then eat cake, the same applies with carbohydrates and proteins etc. The main thing to remember is to ensure you receive a balanced amount of nutrients throughout your day, and as processed foods contain additives which include sugars and salt to enhance taste, you may find that your intake of these items is reduced, despite eating more desserts.

How Does It Work

By eating clean you are putting only natural food sources into your body eliminating the chemicals and additional added ingredients found in processed foods.

These additives added to the basic ingredients have been found to cause many of the ailments the last few generations regularly suffer from. Consumed occasionally and in small amounts these additives can be processed by the body with minimal adverse effects, however, our current eating habits mean that most of consume excessively high amounts of these ingredients.

So what is in processed food and why is it bad for you?

Sugar (often disguised)
One of the worst offenders in processed food is sugar, often disguised under a variety of names including:

- Agave nectar
- Corn syrup
- Crystalline fructose
- Dextrose,
- Fruit juice concentrates
- Glucose
- Honey
- Sucrose

While sugar improves the flavour of foods and provides a boost to your energy levels it can also have an extremely damaging effect on the metabolism.

Additionally, it can cause insulin resistance leading to diabetes, raise triglyceride to dangerous levels leading to high cholesterol and heart disease and increase the accumulation of fat around and in the liver and abdomen which can result in dangerous levels of obesity.

There are also links to high sugar levels being associated with some forms of cancer.

Refined Carbohydrates
Carbohydrates are a necessary part of our diet as they provide a steady release of energy; however the refined carbohydrates such as those found in processed foods are not healthy. This type of carbohydrate is digested very quickly which leads to spikes and dips in blood sugar and affects our insulin levels.

These spikes and dips can lead to both short and long term health problems and have an adverse affect on our emotional stability causing unnatural highs and lows in mood.

Fats

Processed foods often contain refined or hydrogenated vegetable or seed oils which, when consumed, convert to Trans fats. Because these fats are labelled simply as a vegetable or seed oil the damaging effects of them is often overlooked. High levels of these harmful fats can lead to heart disease, body inflammation and oxidation.

Additives

Not all chemicals are required to be listed on the ingredients list of a product and as many are listed with a long, unpronounceable name or a simple code using letters and numbers, most of us do not question them.

The four main categories for additives are:

- **Colorants:** These are chemicals which are added to provide specific colours to the food and used to improve the look of processed foods to entice you to buy them.
- **Preservatives:** Chemicals added to increase the longevity of food before it starts to rot.
- **Flavorings:** Chemicals added to improve the flavour
- **Texturants:** Chemicals which are added to give or improve the texture of food.

One example of a preservative found in bread is **Ammonium Sulphate** and is considered harmless in small amounts. But how much bread or bread products do you consume.

This ingredient sounds innocuous until you consider what it is: Ammonium Sulphate is a chemical combination of Sulphur, Nitrogen, Hydrogen and Oxygen and it is primarily used as a fertiliser for soil.

This is just one example of the chemicals that can be used and hidden in your processed foods but there are a whole lot more of them in each product

Just by eliminating these ingredients from your diet you will feel and look healthier, but what about the necessary dietary requirements you are not receiving by eating processed food such as essential nutrients and fibre.

A varied clean diet should provide you with everything you need to maximise your health and improve your physical and mental wellbeing.

Can It Be Maintained

As this way of eating is simply based on eating unprocessed foods, it is easy to maintain. Our ancestors had no access to processed foods and so always ate clean. Unfortunately, food hygiene was not prevalent in times past so the benefits were not as obvious as they are today.

To maintain a clean eating way of life you need only change your mind-set in the approach to food and food shopping.

Whether you choose to eat completely clean or you just wish to reduce your processed food intake, a positive approach to how you wish to eat and a little willpower to resist your previous eating habits is all you will need.
If you wish to take things one step further you can try your hand at growing your own fruits and vegetables.

Is It Suitable for Everyone

Yes. Processed food is not a requirement of our bodies. However, it is worth noting that some people may experience a little sluggishness to start with as your body will be withdrawing from the excessive sugar levels found in processed foods. This soon passes and you will find your natural energy levels will balance out.

Is It Affordable

As with all dietary changes, you will notice some change in spending habits as you adapt to unprocessed foods.

A restocking of herbs, spices and other basic store cupboard ingredients will increase your spend initially but the cost per item is minimal and each item needs replacing only as and when it runs out so over time this cost is negligible.

Buying fresh, real food may seem to cost you more but in reality this is rarely the case, and the cost to your future health will be priceless

![Assorted fresh fruits and vegetables arranged in a circular image]

How to Eat Clean

When you first switch to a clean diet it can be difficult to understand which foods are clean foods and which ones are not. When buying fresh foods always aim for the organic varieties, but if this is not possible then any fresh food is better than the processed option.

To help you plan your food shopping, the following lists show a variety of clean foods which you can incorporate into your meal plans.

Fresh Fruit & Vegetables
- All varieties of fresh fruit and vegetables, including raw, frozen fruit and vegetables should be incorporated into your clean diet to ensure a good variety of natural vitamins and minerals. If possible buy organic produce as it is free from pesticides.
- Although most fruits contain sugar, this is a natural sugar and far healthier than the refined sugars found in processed foods.

Meat & Fish
All types of meat and fish are suitable for a clean diet but there are a few guidelines you should be aware of.
- **Beef:** This is best to buy directly from a butcher as you should choose only grass fed and humanely raised beef.
- **Pork:** The majority of pork products are processed so avoid ham and cheaper cuts of pork, gammon and bacon. Stick to only the high quality pork options. Again, a butcher's is the best place to purchase pork as you can gain information as to its quality.
- **Fish:** Always buy fish that has been caught sustainably and limit high mercury content fish to 2 servings per week.

High mercury content fish includes:
- King Mackerel
- Marlin
- Shark
- Swordfish
- Tuna

Poultry & Eggs

All eggs and poultry are a good source of protein but choose the free range, organic options whenever possible.

Many of the cheaper super store varieties of fresh chicken will have added water which cannot be considered as a clean food.

Check for products that state no added water or even salt!

Dairy Products

As with meat, dairy products should be included in your diet but follow these guidelines and remember that any low fat dairy products are processed with a sugar content that would give a candy bar a run for its money!

- **Milk:** Always choose full fat varieties and stick to organic milk whenever possible. For a clean alternative you could switch to pure, unsweetened, organic coconut milk, canned varieties not cartons, or unsweetened organic soy milk.
- **Cheese:** Block cheeses only and full fat varieties. Never buy pre-shredded cheeses or low fat version and stick to the better quality cheeses.
- **Cottage Cheese:** Only good quality, full fat varieties.
- **Yoghurt:** Full fat plain yoghurts. If you prefer flavored yoghurt mix a little whole or pureed fruit into the plain yoghurt.

Beans, Pulses & Seeds

All beans, lentils, chickpeas etc can be included in recipes

For a little variety to your recipes try adding sunflower, flax or sesame seeds.

Unrefined Grains
- **Wheat:** Use wholemeal varieties of bread, pasta and rice. If possible, stick to organic.
- **Oats:** Use unflavoured rolled oats or steel cut oats in recipes.
- **Flour:** Always use whole wheat flours when cooking and for an alternative to wheat you can use unprocessed coconut or almond flour.

Nuts:

Ensure the packet contains 100% nuts with no additives. Avoid salted or flavoured nuts as these will contain many unnatural ingredients.

Canned Goods

Not all canned goods are unclean but it is best to avoid them when possible. If you need to purchase canned goods ensure you choose no added sugar and low sodium options when possible.

Tinned tomatoes can be a great addition to the kitchen store cupboard. However only choose the varieties that contain no added ingredients.

Cooking Oils

Choose natural oils such as Olive Oil, Coconut oil, and Avocado Oil.

Herbs & Spices

Always choose fresh or dried herbs and spices and avoid seasoning packets. I would recommend in spending a little time and money stocking a great herbs and spice store at home. They will come in so handy when preparing clean meals.

Natural Sweeteners

- **Honey:** Organic when possible
- **Pure syrup:** Avoid the processed bottles and buy organic where possible.

Condiments

Always choose no added sugar varieties

- **Ketchup & Mustard:** It is possible for purchase clean varieties but these are often very difficult to find. The cleanest option is to make your own.

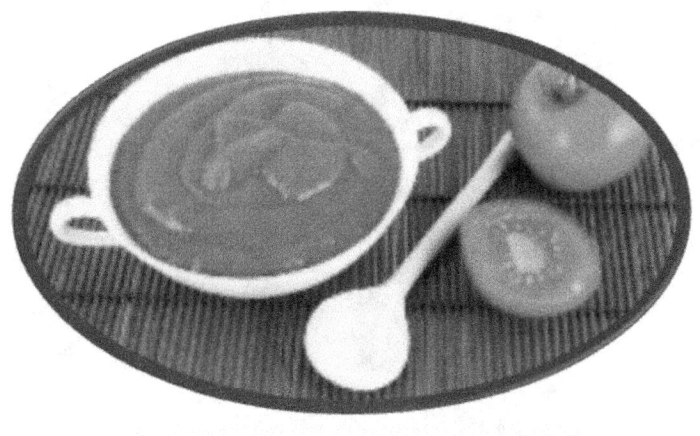

Conversion Tables & Nutrition

Cooking Conversion Tables

Dry Measures

WEIGHT	GRAMS
1 TSP	5
1 TBSP	14
1 OZ	28
1 CUP	227
1 LB	454
1/2 oz.	15g
1 oz.	30g
2 oz.	60g
3 oz.	90g
4 oz.	110g
5 oz.	140g
6 oz.	170g
7 oz.	200g
8 oz.	225g
9 oz.	255g
10 oz.	280g
11 oz.	310g
12 oz.	340g
1 lb	450g

Liquid Measurements

Metric	Imperial	US cups
250ml	8 fl oz.	1 cup
180ml	6 fl oz.	3/4 cup
150ml	5 fl oz.	2/3 cup
120ml	4 fl oz.	1/2 cup
75ml	2 1/2 fl oz.	1/3 cup
60ml	2 fl oz.	1/4 cup
30ml	1 fl oz.	1/8 cup
15ml	1/2 fl oz.	1 tablespoon

Oven Temperature Guide

°C	Gas	°F
110	1/4	225
120/130	1/2	250
140	1	275
150	2	300
160/170	3	325
180	4	350
190	5	375
200/210	6	400
220	7	425
230	8	450
240	9	475

Nutrition

Recommended Daily Allowances

Calculated for adults and children over 4 years of age and based on a daily calorie intake of 2000 calories

Fat	65 grams
Saturated Fatty Acids	20 grams
Protein	50 grams
Carbohydrate	300 grams
Fibre	25 grams

Recipes

This section has been broken down into meal categories to make it easier for your conversion to clean cooking. For those of us not used to real cooking it can be difficult to transfer to making real home cooked meals so have fun with it and once you have become comfortable with these recipes, play around with them and adapt them to suit your palette. Not only will this let you put your own stamp on mealtimes but it will offer you a greater variety from the same recipes.

Breakfast

Sweet Potato Pancakes

Serves 1

Ingredients:
2 eggs
1 medium sweet potato, (baked)
Pinch of allspice
Pinch of cinnamon
1tsp olive oil
½ cup plain yoghurt
1 tsp pure maple syrup

Directions:
1. Remove skin from sweet potato and mash the flesh
2. Whisk together 2 eggs
3. Stir a pinch of cinnamon and allspice into the whisked egg
4. Stir egg mixture into mashed sweet potato until blended together well
5. Divide into 3 or 4 portions
6. Heat olive oil in a frying pan over a medium to high heat
7. Pour one portion of potato batter into frying pan and cook for 5 or 6 minutes
8. Using a spatula, turn over the pancake and cook for a further 4 to 5 minutes
9. Mix together plain yoghurt and maple syrup
10. Remove pancake from pan, drizzle with yoghurt dressing and serve

Nutritional Information
Calories: 336
Fat: 11.7g
Protein: 24.7 g
Carbohydrate: 32.83g
Fibre: 4.9g

Seasoned Omelette with Tomatoes & Spring Onion

Serves 1

Ingredients:
4 eggs
¼ cup diced tomato
2 spring onions, finely chopped
¼ tsp mustard seeds
Pinch of turmeric
Pinch of black pepper
½ tsp salt
1 tbsp olive oil

Directions:
1. Whisk together eggs & add salt
2. Heat oil in a frying pan over a medium to high heat and add mustard seeds and turmeric, (note: mustard seeds will pop as they cook) and fry for 30 seconds stirring continuously
3. Add onions and cook for a further 30 seconds, stirring continuously
4. Add tomatoes and continue to stir for a further 1 minute
5. Pour egg mixture into frying pan and cook until edges begin to set
6. Reduce heat to low and continue to cook. (Gently tease the edge of omelette away from the pan to avoid sticking)
7. When centre of omelette is almost completely set, remove from heat and place under a medium grill to finish cooking and brown the top
8. Sprinkle with black pepper and serve

Nutritional Information
Calories: 216
Fat: 16.9g
Protein: 13.3g
Carbohydrate: 3.4g
Fibre: 0.9g

Avocado Toast with Egg

Serves 2

Ingredients:
4 eggs
1 avocado, peeled, cooked & mashed
4 slices whole wheat bread
¼ tsp salt
¼ tsp pepper
1 tbsp olive oil
½ cup fresh salsa

Directions:
1. Toast the bread
2. Heat oil in a frying pan over a medium to high heat
3. Crack eggs into frying pan and fry until cooked
4. Divide mashed avocado into 4 portions and spread onto toast, one portion per slice
5. Place 1 fried egg onto each slice of toast
6. Sprinkle with salt and pepper
7. Drizzle each slice with salsa and serve

Nutritional Information
Calories: 247
Fat: 14.5g
Protein: 11g
Carbohydrate: 19g
Fibre: 6g

Pancakes

Serves 2 (3 pancakes per person)

Ingredients:
2 large eggs
2 medium bananas
4 tbsp whole wheat flour
Olive oil

Directions:
1. Whisk eggs
2. Fold in the flour and whisk until smooth
3. Mash banana
4. Stir batter into the banana and mix till as smooth as possible
5. Heat oil in frying pan over a medium to high heat
6. Spoon batter for 1 pancake into frying pan and cook for around 2 minutes or until mixture starts to bubble
7. Flip pancake and cook for a further 1 to 2 minutes until browned
8. Remove from heat and serve with fruit or syrup of choice

Nutritional Information
Calories: 233
Fat: 5.3g
Protein: 9g
Carbohydrate: 39g
Fibre: 3.5g

Spinach & Mushroom Omelette

Serves 3 – 4

Ingredients:
8 medium or large eggs
6 oz baby leaf spinach, chopped
8 oz mushrooms, sliced
½ cup chopped onion
Pinch of thyme
1 clove garlic, finely chopped
¾ tsp salt
¼ tsp pepper
2 tbsp olive oil

Directions:
1. Heat oil in frying pan over a medium to high heat
2. Add onions, garlic, mushrooms and thyme to pan and cook for 5 – 7 minutes
3. Add spinach and cook for a further 4 minutes
4. Whisk eggs
5. Whisk salt & pepper into eggs and pour mixture into frying pan, reduce heat to medium
6. Cook until edges begin to set
7. Reduce heat to low and continue to cook. (Gently tease the edge of omelette away from the pan to avoid sticking)
8. When centre of omelette is almost completely set, remove from heat and place under a medium grill to finish cooking and brown the top
9. Sprinkle with black pepper, divide into 4 and serve

Nutritional Information
Calories: 244
Fat: 16g
Protein: 16g
Carbohydrate: 11g
Fibre: 3g

Rolled Oats with Almond & Blueberry

Serves 2

Ingredients:
1 cup rolled oats
1 cup milk
4 tbsp toasted almonds
1 cup blueberries, (or berries of choice)

Directions:
1. Bring milk to the boil and stir in rolled oats
2. Reduce heat and simmer for 5 to 8 minutes until oats are cooked
3. Remove from heat & place oats into 2 bowls
4. Sprinkle with almonds and berries
5. Serve hot or cold

Nutritional Information
Calories: 306
Fat: 9g
Protein: 14g
Carbohydrate: 46g
Fibre: 7g

Spiced Quinoa

Serves 1

Ingredients:
½ cup quinoa, rinsed well
1 cup milk
1 cup water
½ tsp cinnamon
Pinch of nutmeg
Pinch of ginger
Pinch of salt
1 tbsp olive oil
½ tsp vanilla extract
1 large egg white
2 tbsp raisins
2 tbsp honey

Directions:
1. Heat oil in a frying pan over a medium to high heat and add quinoa
2. Cook quinoa, stirring continuously for 2 – 4 minutes until grains have separated
3. Bring to the boil then reduce to a low to medium simmer
4. Cook for 20 – 30 minutes until quinoa is soft then remove from heat
5. Stir vanilla extract and honey into quinoa
6. Whisk egg white and add quinoa, 1 tbsp at a time stirring with each addition until fully incorporated together
7. Stir in raisins and return to pan
8. Cook over a medium to high heat for 2 minutes, stirring continuously
9. Remove from heat and serve

Nutritional Information
Calories: 311
Fat: 4g
Protein: 12g
Carbohydrate: 58g
Fibre: 4g

Lunch

Fennel, Spinach & Shrimp Salad

Serves 4

Ingredients:
½ cup red onion, finely sliced
2 tbsp finely chopped white onion
1 cup cherry tomatoes, halved
3 rashers bacon
9oz baby leaf spinach
1lb jumbo shrimp, deveined and peeled
1 medium fennel bulb, finely sliced
1 tsp Dijon mustard
1 tbsp balsamic vinegar
3 tbsp extra virgin olive oil
¼ tsp salt
¼ tsp black pepper

Directions:
1. Heat oil in a frying pan over a medium heat
2. Roughly chop bacon and add to frying pan. Cook until crispy and remove from pan. Retain the oil in frying pan
3. Add shrimp to pan and fry for 2 minutes, tossing shrimp occasionally
4. Remove from heat and set aside
5. In a large bowl mix together cooked bacon, red onion, fennel, tomatoes and baby leaf spinach
6. In a separate bowl, mix together the remaining unused ingredients then stir in the shrimp
7. Mix salad and oil mixtures together and toss lightly before serving

Nutritional Information
Calories: 274; Fat: 13.5g; Protein: 27.5g; Carbohydrate: 11.2g;
Fibre: 3.5g

Spinach & Feta Quiche

Serves 4

Crust Ingredients:
2 cup quinoa, (cooked)
1 large egg
Pinch of black pepper

Filling Ingredients:
½ onion, finely sliced
5 oz baby leaf spinach, chopped
½ cup milk
4 large eggs
2 large egg whites
1½ oz feta cheese, crumbled
¼ tsp crushed red pepper
¼ tsp ground black pepper
½ tsp salt
1 tsp olive oil

Crust Directions:
1. Preheat oven to 375°c
2. Whisk egg and stir together cooked quinoa, egg and pepper
3. Grease a 9"quiche dish and press quinoa mixture into base and sides
4. Bake for 20 minutes and allow to cool

Filling Directions:
1. Heat oil in a frying pan over a medium heat
2. Add onions and cook for 3 minutes
3. Add spinach and cook for a further 3 minutes
4. Remove from heat and allow to cool
5. Whisk together eggs and egg whites
6. Whisk in milk, red pepper, black pepper and salt
7. Spread spinach and onion mix over the baked quinoa base
8. Pour egg mixture into the quiche base and sprinkle with feta cheese
9. Return to oven and bake for 35 minutes

Nutritional Information
Calories: 282
Fat: 11.6g
Protein: 17g
Carbohydrate: 28g
Fibre: 5g

Quinoa Salad

Serves 8

Salad Ingredients:
2 tbsp finely diced red onion
½ cup finely diced onion
5 dates, pitted and chopped
½ lb cooked asparagus, roughly chopped
1 cup quinoa, uncooked
2 cups water
1 large orange, peeled and segmented
¼ cup chopped, roasted pecans
½ jalapeno pepper, deseeded and finely chopped
½ tsp salt
1 tsp olive oil

Dressing Ingredients:
1 clove garlic, finely chopped
2 tbsp fresh mint, finely chopped
2 tbsp freshly squeezed lemon juice
¼ tsp salt
¼ tsp pepper
1 tbsp extra virgin olive oil

Salad Directions:
1. Add oil to a frying pan and heat over a medium to high heat
2. Add white onions and fry for 2 minutes
3. Add quinoa and fry, stirring regularly, for a further 5 minutes
4. Add water and salt to frying pan and bring to a boil
5. Reduce heat and simmer for 15 minutes
6. Remove from heat and allow to cool until water is absorbed, usually around 10 to 15 minutes
7. Transfer to a large bowl and add the remaining salad ingredients
8. Toss gently to combine ingredients

Dressing Directions:
1. Mix all ingredients together, except mint
2. Drizzle over salad
3. Garnish with mint and serve

Nutritional Information
Calories: 164
Fat: 6.3g
Protein: 4.3g
Carbohydrate: 24.7g
Fibre: 3.4g

Spicy Sweet Potato Soup

Serves 4

Crust Ingredients:
1 onion, diced
2 cloves garlic, finely chopped
1 large sweet potato, peeled and diced
¼ cup shredded coconut
15 fl.oz coconut milk
¼ cup chopped, fresh coriander
2 tbsp coconut oil
Juice of 1 lime, freshly squeezed
2 tbsp curry powder
¼ tsp cayenne pepper
½ tsp cumin
½ tsp salt

Directions:
1. Heat coconut oil in a frying pan over a medium heat
2. Add onions and fry until soft
3. Add garlic and cook for a further 1 minute
4. Add sweet potatoes and cook for an additional 5 minutes, stirring occasionally
5. Stir in curry powder, cayenne pepper, cumin and salt and continue cooking for another minute
6. Stir in coconut milk and bring up to a fast simmer
7. Reduce to a low heat and simmer for 20 to 25 minutes
8. Remove from heat and pour into a blend
9. Blend until smooth
10. Pour into a serving dish and stir in lime juice
11. Sprinkle with coconut and coriander to serve

Nutritional Information
Calories: 246
Fat: 18g
Protein: 2g
Carbohydrate: 19g
Fibre: 5g

Vegetable Rice

Serves 4

Ingredients:
1 ¹/₃ cups cooked and cooled brown rice
1 cup cherry tomatoes, halved
1 cup green soybeans, shelled
¼ cup toasted pine nuts
2 cups chopped courgette
3 tbsp freshly squeezed lemon juice
2 tsp lemon zest
½ cup fresh basil, roughly chopped
½ oz fresh parmesan cheese, finely grated
3 tbsp olive oil
1 tsp salt
¼ tsp ground black pepper

Directions:
1. In a large mixing bowl, mix together all ingredients except olive oil, courgette and parmesan
2. Heat 1 tbsp olive oil in a frying pan over a medium to high heat
3. Add courgette and cook for 4 – 5 minutes, stirring occasionally
4. Remove from pan and allow to cool
5. Stir courgette into the remaining 2 tbsp's oil
6. Combine courgette mixture with other ingredients and toss well
7. Sprinkle with parmesan shavings to serve

Nutritional Information
Calories: 305
Fat: 19.1g
Protein: 9.6g
Carbohydrate: 25.4g
Fibre: 4.9g

Baked Sweet Potato

Serves 4

Ingredients:
4 medium sweet potatoes
425g canned chickpeas, rinsed and drained
½ tbsp olive oil
½ tsp cumin
½ tsp coriander
½ tsp paprika
½ tsp cinnamon
½ tsp fresh lemon juice

Sauce Ingredients
¼ cup hummus
3 garlic cloves, finely chopped
1 tsp dill
1 tbsp fresh lemon juice
Unsweetened almond milk, (to thin sauce)

Sauce Directions:
1. Mix together all sauce ingredients, (except almond milk)
2. When fully mixed, slowly add 1 tbsp almond milk at a time and stir well. Continue until sauce is pourable

Directions:

1. Preheat oven to 400°c and line a baking sheet with foil
2. Clean sweet potatoes and halve, lengthways
3. Rub potatoes with a little olive oil and place face down on baking sheet
4. Mix together olive oil, cumin, coriander, paprika, cinnamon and lemon juice and stir in the chickpeas
5. Spread chickpea mixture over the baking sheet and place in over for 45 – 60 minutes
6. Remove from oven and plate up sweet potatoes, 2 halves per serving
7. Sprinkle with chickpea mixture and drizzle over sauce to serve

Nutritional Information

Calories: 313
Fat: 5g
Protein: 8.6g
Carbohydrate: 60g
Fibre: 11.7g

Vegetable Pasta & Prawns with Avocado Dressing

Serves 1

Ingredients:
3 small courgettes
5 oz cooked prawns, deveined and peeled
½ cup cherry tomatoes, halved
2 cups water

Dressing Ingredients:
¼ avocado
1 garlic clove, finely chopped
½ cup fresh chopped basil
Juice of ¼ lemon
Pinch salt & pepper

Dressing Directions:
1. Place garlic, lemon juice, salt, pepper, basil and avocado into a blender
2. Blend until almost smooth

Directions:
1. Peel courgettes and slice into long, thin strips, (like thick spaghetti)
2. Bring water to boil and blanche courgette strips for 30 seconds
3. Remove from boiling water and rinse in cold water then set to one side
4. In a large mixing bowl, place courgettes, prawns, cherry tomatoes and dressing and stir together well
5. Press quinoa mixture into base and sides of quiche dish

Nutritional Information
Calories: 224
Fat: 5.9g
Protein: 26.3g
Carbohydrate: 20.6g
Fibre: 8.5g

Dinner

Lemon Chicken Kebabs

Serves 2

Ingredients:
6oz boneless, skinless chicken breast, chopped into 1 ½" pieces
1 cup cherry tomatoes, chopped
3 tbsp fresh lemon juice
1 tbsp garlic, finely chopped
1½ tsp oregano
¾ tsp salt
¾ tsp ground black pepper
2 cups fresh parsley
3 tbsp extra virgin olive oil

Directions:
1. In a small bowl, mix together 2 tbsp lemon juice, 2 tsp chopped garlic, 1 tsp oregano, ½ tsp salt, ½ tsp pepper and 1 tbsp olive oil
2. Add chicken and stir well
3. Leave to marinate in refrigerator for 2 – 4 hours
4. Remove chicken from bowl and divide into 4 portions
5. Thread each portion onto 1 or 2 skewers
6. Cook under a grill or on a griddle, turning regularly until fully cooked, usually around 6 to 10 minutes
7. Mix together remaining ingredients, excluding parsley, and whisk together well
8. Drizzle over cooked kebabs and garnish with parsley

Nutritional Information
Calories: 311
Fat: 14.9g
Protein: 38g
Carbohydrate: 6g
Fibre: 2g

Beef with Red Onion Marmalade

Serves 2

Ingredients:
4 x 4oz beef steaks, 1" thick
1 large red onion, sliced into rings
2 tbsp honey
2 tbsp red wine vinegar
1 tsp thyme
½ tsp salt
¼ tsp ground black pepper
1 tbsp olive oil

Directions:
1. Heat oil in a large frying pan over a medium to high heat
2. Add onion and cook for 3 minutes
3. Add vinegar, honey and ¼ tsp salt to pan and reduce heat
4. Simmer, stirring occasionally for 7 to 9 minutes until thickened slightly and remove from heat
5. Turn grill on high
6. Mix together remaining salt, pepper and thyme with a little olive oil and rub over beef
7. Cook steaks under the grill for 4 to 6 minutes each side
8. Serve with onion mixture and a choice of potatoes, salad or both

Nutritional Information
Calories: 289
Fat: 11.4g
Protein: 32.5g
Carbohydrate: 12.6g
Fibre: 0.8g

Greek Fish

Serves 2

Ingredients:
5 small potatoes, cleaned and sliced into wedges
1 onion, sliced
2 cloves garlic, roughly chopped
2 fresh cod or white fish fillets, de-skinned, around 100g each
2 large tomatoes, cut into wedges
½ lemon, cut into wedges
2 tbsp olive oil
½ tsp dried oregano
Fresh parsley, roughly chopped to garnish

Directions:
1. Preheat oven to 200°c
2. Mix together olive oil, garlic and oregano
3. Toss potato wedges and onion in mixture and spread onto a baking tray
4. Bake for 30 minutes, turning half way through cooking
5. Add lemon and tomatoes and cook for a further 10 minutes
6. Place fish fillets on top and continue to cook for a further 10 to 15 minutes until fish is cooked through
7. Sprinkle with parsley and serve

Nutritional Information
Calories: 388
Fat: 13g
Protein: 23g
Carbohydrate: 42g
Fibre: 6g

Lentil & Aubergine Bake

Serves 4

Ingredients:
2 aubergines, sliced lengthways, ½ cm thick
140g lentils
2 onions, finely chopped
3 garlic cloves, finely chopped
300g butternut squash, cooked
400g chopped tomato
125g mozzarella, torn
3 tbsp extra virgin olive oil
Small handful fresh basil, chopped
Pinch of salt & pepper
½ cup water

Directions:
1. Preheat oven to 200°c
2. Using 2 tbsp olive oil, brush aubergines slices, (both sides) with olive oil and spread onto a baking tray
3. Sprinkle with salt & pepper and bake for 15 to 20 minutes
4. Cook lentils, (follow instructions on packet)
5. Heat 1 tbsp olive oil in a large frying pan over a medium to high heat
6. Add onions & garlic and cook for 2 to 3 minutes
7. Stir in squash, tomatoes and water and simmer for 10 to 15 minutes until thickened
8. Stir in lentils, basil and another pinch of salt & pepper then remove from heat
9. Spread a layer of lentil mixture into a small baking dish and top with aubergine slices
10. Continue to layer in this way until all mixture and aubergines have been used
11. Sprinkle with mozzarella and bake for a further 15 minutes

Nutritional Information
Calories:359;   Fat:16g;   Protein:19g;   Carbohydrate:34g;
Fibre:10g

Courgette & Tomato Stew

Serves 4

Ingredients:
3 courgettes, cut into chunks
1 onion, roughly chopped
2 garlic bulbs, finely chopped
800g canned chopped tomatoes
25g parmesan, grated
1 tbsp olive oil
1 bunch fresh basil, torn

Directions:
1. In a large frying pan, heat olive oil over a medium heat
2. Add onions and cook until they begin to brown, (5 to 10 minutes)
3. Add garlic and cook for a further 5 minutes, stirring occasionally
4. Add courgettes and cook for an additional 5 minutes
5. Stir in tomatoes and bring to a fast boil
6. Reduce heat and simmer for 35 to 40 minutes
7. Stir in parmesan and basil
8. Remove from heat and serve

Nutritional Information
Calories: 114
Fat: 5g
Protein: 6g
Carbohydrate: 10g
Fibre: 3g

Chana Masala

Serves 2

Ingredients:
1 medium onion, chopped
1 clove garlic, finely chopped
75g quick cook basmati rice, brown
400g canned chopped tomatoes
400g canned chickpeas, drained and rinsed
220g baby leaf spinach
1cm ginger, peeled and grated
Juice of half a lemon
½ red chilli pepper, deseeded and finely chopped
1 tbsp extra virgin olive oil
1 tsp cumin seed
1 tsp ground coriander
1 tsp cumin
1 tsp paprika
1 tsp garam masala
1 tsp turmeric
200ml water

Directions:
1. Cook rice and set aside
2. Place cumin seeds into a large frying pan and heat, (no oil), over a medium heat until popped. Remove from pan and set aside
3. Add oil to the frying pan and heat
4. Add onion, ginger, chilli and garlic and cook for 3 minutes
5. Reduce to low heat and stir in garam masala, turmeric, coriander, cumin and paprika and cook for 2 minutes
6. Stir in tomatoes, chickpeas and water
7. Increase heat and bring to the boil before reducing to a simmer for 10 minutes
8. Stir in lemon juice and spinach the remove from the heat
9. Serve over brown rice

Nutritional Information
Calories: 420
Fat: 12g
Protein: 20g
Carbohydrate: 60g
Fibre: 12g

Salmon & Salsa Salad

Serves 2

Ingredients:
2 salmon fillets
1 clove garlic, finely chopped
Juice of 1 lime
    (using same lime, grate zest then quarter)
1 tsp chilli powder
½ tsp ground coriander
¼ tsp cumin
2 tsp olive oil

Salsa Ingredients:
1 red onion, finely chopped
1 clove garlic, finely chopped
1 avocado, peeled, de-stoned and chopped
1 corn on the cob
1 red bell pepper, deseeded and finely chopped
1 red chilli, halved, deseeded and finely chopped
Handful of fresh coriander, finely chopped

Salmon Directions:

1. In a small bowl, mix together garlic, 1 tsp lime juice, olive oil, cumin, coriander and chilli powder
2. Rub mixture into both sides of salmon fillets
3. Heat a little oil in a frying pan over a medium heat
4. Cook salmon fillets for 2 minutes per side
5. Serve with salsa salad

Salsa Directions:

1. Boil corn on the cob for around 7 to 8 minutes until soft
2. Remove corn from the cob and place in a large mixing bowl
3. Add remaining lime juice, lime zest, red onion, garlic, avocado, chilli and bell pepper and stir together
4. To serve, add lime wedges and sprinkle with fresh coriander

Nutritional Information

Calories: 530
Fat: 32g
Protein: 29g
Carbohydrate: 27g
Fibre: 9g

Snacks

Honey & Almond Bar

8 Bars

Ingredients:
¼ cup chopped almonds
¼ cup sunflower seeds
1 cup rolled oats
1 tbsp golden flax seeds
1 cup unsweetened puffed rice, (cereal)
¼ cup turbinado sugar, (this is a minimally refined sugar)
¼ cup almond butter, (creamed)
¼ cup honey
1 tbsp sesame seeds
$1/_3$ cup currants
$1/_3$ cup dried almonds, (chopped)
$1/_3$ cup raisins
½ tsp vanilla extract
Pinch salt

Directions:

1. Preheat oven to 180°c and grease or line an 8" square baking tray
2. Mix together sunflower seeds, sesame seeds, flax seeds and oats and spread over a flat baking tray
3. Bake for 20 minutes, shaking tray after 10 minutes
4. Add puffed rice cereal, apricots, currants and raisins to a mixing bowl and stir in baked seeds and oats
5. In a small saucepan, mix together honey, sugar, almond butter, vanilla and salt
6. Heat saucepan over a low to medium heat for 3 to 5 minutes until bubbles appear, stirring regularly
7. Pour honey mixture into mixing bowl and stir to combine all ingredients
8. Transfer to prepared 8" baking tray and spread evenly. Press mixture down firmly
9. Allow to cool for at least 30 to 60 minutes
10. Slice into bars and serve

Nutritional Information
Calories: 244
Fat: 10g
Protein: 5g
Carbohydrate: 38g
Fibre: 3g

Strawberry & Banana Muffins

12 Muffins

Ingredients:
1 large egg
2 ripe bananas, mashed
½ cup plain yoghurt
½ cup unsweetened almond milk
1¼ cup whole wheat flour
½ cup, naturally sweetened, whey protein powder, vanilla flavour
2 tbsp flax seeds
2 tsp vanilla extract
2 tsp baking powder
1 cup, chopped fresh strawberries
Pinch salt
Spray oil or butter to grease muffin tray

Directions:
1. Preheat oven to 180°c and grease or line muffin tray
2. Whisk egg and add yoghurt, almond milk, mashed banana and vanilla extract
3. In a separate bowl, mix together flour, protein powder, baking powder, salt and flax seeds
4. Add dry ingredients mixture to the wet mixture and fold together to combine
5. Gently stir in strawberries
6. Distribute evenly between muffin moulds
7. Bake for 18 to 20 minutes until fully cooked
8. Allow to cool before serving

Nutritional Information
Calories: 100
Fat: 1.5g
Protein: 8.4g
Carbohydrate: 16g
Fibre: 3g

Berry Parfait

Serves 2

Ingredients:
1 cup oats
½ cup almonds, chopped
3 tbsp pure coconut oil
½ tsp cinnamon
2 cups plain yoghurt
½ cup blueberries
½ cup blackberries
½ cup raspberries

Directions:
1. Preheat oven to 180°c and line a baking sheet
2. In a small saucepan, heat coconut oil over a low heat until liquid
3. Add oats, cinnamon and almonds to saucepan and stir well until ingredients have combined
4. Spread mixture evenly over the baking tray and bake for 20 minutes, stirring halfway
5. Remove from oven and allow to cool
6. Layer granola mix, yoghurt and berries alternately in a dessert glass and serve

Nutritional Information
Calories: 244
Fat: 10g
Protein: 5g
Carbohydrate: 38g
Fibre: 3g

Energising Smoothie

Serves 3

Ingredients:
1 small banana, sliced then frozen
1 cup baby leaf spinach
1 cup frozen, unsweetened blackberries or raspberries
½ cup plain yoghurt
½ cup pure pomegranate juice
½" piece of ginger, chopped
1 cup cold, unsweetened green tea
1 cup crushed ice

Directions:
1. Add all ingredients to a blender and blend until smooth. If too thick, add a little more green tea

Nutritional Information
Calories: 131
Fat: 1g
Protein: 7g
Carbohydrate: 26g
Fibre: 4g

Mango Dessert

Serves 2

Ingredients:
½ frozen banana, sliced
½ cup frozen mango
½ frozen pineapple
$^1/_3$ cup unsweetened coconut milk
2 cups plain yoghurt
½ cup blueberries
½ cup blackberries
½ cup raspberries

Topping Ingredients:
2 tbsp pomegranate seeds
¼ cup fresh chopped pineapple
1 tbsp unsweetened coconut flakes

Directions:
1. Add coconut milk, banana, pineapple and mango to a blender and blend until smooth
2. Pour into a bowl and sprinkle with toppings

Nutritional Information
Calories: 240
Fat: 4g
Protein: 3.3g
Carbohydrate: 53.9g
Fibre: 7.8g

Conclusion

Thank you for buying this book and I hope you have enjoyed reading it as much as I enjoyed writing it.

Now you understand the rules of clean eating, the next step is to plan your meals and get cooking. All the recipes are easy to prepare and cook and in a short time you will be providing your family with healthy meals that not only taste and look great, but will improve their overall mental and physical health.

Why not try out your new cooking skills on friends and extended family. These recipes will make you the toast of any party.

Finally, if you have enjoyed this book, please leave a review so that others can benefit from the information included within it.

Thank you and good luck.